Marwa Gragouri
Héla Gargouri
Ahmed Tlili

Study of rabies knowledge and prevention measures

Marwa Gragouri
Héla Gargouri
Ahmed Tlili

Study of rabies knowledge and prevention measures

Study of nurses' and bite victims' knowledge of rabies and preventive measures

ScienciaScripts

Cover image: www.ingimage.com

This book is a translation from the original published under ISBN 978-620-6-71368-5.

Publisher:
Sciencia Scripts
is a trademark of
Dodo Books Indian Ocean Ltd. and OmniScriptum S.R.L publishing group

120 High Road, East Finchley, London, N2 9ED, United Kingdom
Str. Armeneasca 28/1, office 1, Chisinau MD-2012, Republic of Moldova, Europe
Printed at: see last page
ISBN: 978-620-7-70439-2

STUDY OF THE KNOWLEDGE OF NURSES AND VICTIMS OF ANIMAL BITES WITH REGARD TO RABIES: PREVENTIVE MEASURES

DIRECTED BY :
DR. MARWA GARGOURI
AHU IN INFECTIOUS DISEASES
CHU MOHAMED BEN SASSI DE GABES MAIL: MARWAGARGOURI.INFECTIEUX@GMAIL.COM

CONTENTS

INTRODUCTION

Rabies is a vaccine-preventable viral zoonosis that affects the central nervous system. As soon as clinical symptoms appear, rabies is fatal in almost 100% of cases. Domestic dogs are responsible for transmitting the rabies virus to humans in almost 99% of cases. However, rabies affects both domestic and wild animals. It is spread to humans and animals through saliva, usually by bites, scratches or direct contact with mucous membranes (e.g. eyes, mouth or open wounds). [1]

The introduction of a National Rabies Control Programme (PNLR) in 1982 led to a significant reduction in human rabies, which was made possible by the fact that rabies is a notifiable disease in Tunisia [2].However, as a result of a decline in the activities of the PNLR, particularly in its vaccination and stray dog control components, an upsurge in cases of human rabies was recorded from 1990 onwards, with an epidemiological peak in 1992, when 25 cases of human rabies were reported. This situation prompted the country's health authorities to relaunch the campaign [3].

In 2021, we recorded 2 cases of death due to human rabies, which means that nurses' knowledge of rabies needs to be reassessed, as does the quality of care provided to people attacked by animals that transmit this disease. We also need to process the information acquired from the victim population on the basics to know about rabies in terms of what to do, which can influence a well-defined care pathway. In addition, it is essential to be able to count on multi-sectoral participation and collaboration as part of the "One World, One Health" approach, which encompasses community education, awareness programmes and vaccination campaigns, and emphasises the responsibility of both partners for better prevention.

The objectives of our work are :

✓ Study nurses' knowledge of rabies.

✓ Improving care techniques and treatment modalities for rabies in the emergency department

✓ Studying the knowledge of bite victims

on the seriousness of their situation if they do not take the necessary precautions.

in charge.

✓ Suggest measures to prevent complications from bites.

I. QUESTIONNAIRE MATERIALS AND METHODS

1. Search quote :

This is a descriptive study involving the hospital's healthcare staff. university hospital, the military hospital and the basic health care centres in Gabès. In the course of this study, the members interviewed answered our questionnaire personally and anonymously.

2. Study environment and period :

This study was carried out at the university hospital, the military hospital and the basic health care centres in Gabès during the months of February and March 2023.For hospitals, the departments included in our study were the following:

- ► Gabès Military Hospital Emergency Department
- ► Gabès University Hospital Emergency Department
- ► Department of Infectious Diseases, Gabès University Hospital

3. The study population :

In this study, we selected a population of 80 healthcare workers in the following health establishments:

- ❖Gabès University Hospital Emergency Department: 21
- ❖Gabès military hospital emergency department: 9
- ❖Department of Infectious Diseases, University Hospital, London

Gabès: 11

- ❖CSSB Tbelbou: 4
- ❖CSSB Wassit: 7
- ❖CSSB Kattena: 8
- ❖CSSB Cité Al'Amal: 6
- ❖CSSB Manara: 3
- ❖CSSB Ghanouch: 5
- ❖CSSB Bouchamma: 6

4. Inclusion and non-inclusion criteria :

4.1. Inclusion criteria :

- ❖ Staff working in emergency departments and basic healthcare centres.
- ❖ The staff who were present when our survey was carried out.
- ❖ The staff who agreed to answer our questions.

4.2. Non-inclusion criteria :

- ❖ Staff working in other departments.
- ❖ The refusal declared by certain healthcare staff.
- ❖ Some staff were absent during our study period.

5. Data collection :

This study was carried out by means of a questionnaire consisting of 21 questions: an identification section containing 5 questions; 3 sections containing 6 open questions and 10 closed questions. We asked 3 questions in the study of nurses' knowledge of an animal bite, 11 questions in the study of the degree of implementation of the rabies control protocol and 2 questions in the study of preventive measures. We targeted 80 health personnel working at the university hospital, the military hospital and the basic health care centres in Gabès.

6. Data collection process :

We were present in the departments concerned to inform potential employees about the study (context and objectives). We then distributed the questionnaire to those who agreed to take part. It took each staff member an average of 15 minutes to answer the various parts of the questionnaire.

7. Data capture and analysis :

The data was collected manually. Data entry was carried out using computer equipment (2 computers) typed in Microsoft Office Word 2010 and processed using Microsoft Office Excel 2010. The results are represented using Excel and Word.

II. MATERIALS AND METHODS FOR THE VICTIM QUESTIONNAIRE

1. Search quote :

This is a descriptive study including animal bite victims distributed to different basic health care centres in Gabès: Tbelbou, Wassit, Kattena, cité Al'Amal, Manara, Ghanouch. We also included victims seen in the emergency department of Gabès University Hospital. In the course of this study, the members interviewed answered our questionnaire personally and anonymously.

2. Study environment and period :

This study was carried out at the University Hospital of Gabès and the basic health care centres during the two months of February and March 2023. The departments included in our study were the following:

- ► The emergency department
- ► Basic healthcare centres

3. The study population :

In this study, we included a population of 75 victims of animal bites in the emergency departments of the University Hospital of Gabès and the basic health care centres.

- ❖Gabes University Hospital Emergency Department: 31
- ❖CSSB Tbelbou: 5
- ❖CSSB Wassit: 17
- ❖CSSB Kattena: 8
- ❖CSSB quoted Al'Amal : 6
- ❖CSSB Manara: 3
- ❖CSSB Ghanouch: 5

4. Inclusion and non-inclusion criteria :

4.1. Inclusion criteria :

- ✓ Age >18
- ✓ Patient consent

4.2. Criteria for non-inclusion :

✓ Age <18

✓ Refusal to take part in the study

✓ Disability mental making impossible to collect all necessary information.

5. Data collection :

This study was carried out by means of a questionnaire consisting of 18 questions: an identification part comprising 6 questions, a second part of 12 questions (containing 3 open questions and 9 closed questions) for the study of the knowledge of rabies among victims of animal bites, targeting victims at the university hospital and basic healthcare centres in Gabès.

6. Data collection process :

We were present in the relevant departments to inform potential victims about the study (context and objectives). We then distributed the questionnaire to those who agreed to take part. Each person took an average of 10 minutes to answer the various parts of the questionnaire.

7. Data capture and analysis :

The data was collected manually. Data entry was carried out using computer equipment (2 computers) typed in Microsoft Office Word 2010 and processed using Microsoft Office Excel 2010. The results were represented using Excel and Word.

III. ANALYSIS AND RESULTS OF PERSONNEL QUESTIONNAIRE

During our study period, 80 healthcare workers were included.

A. socio-demographic data

1. Breakdown of staff by gender :

We found that the majority of the population studied was female (54%), with a sex ratio (M/F) of 0.6 (Figure 1).

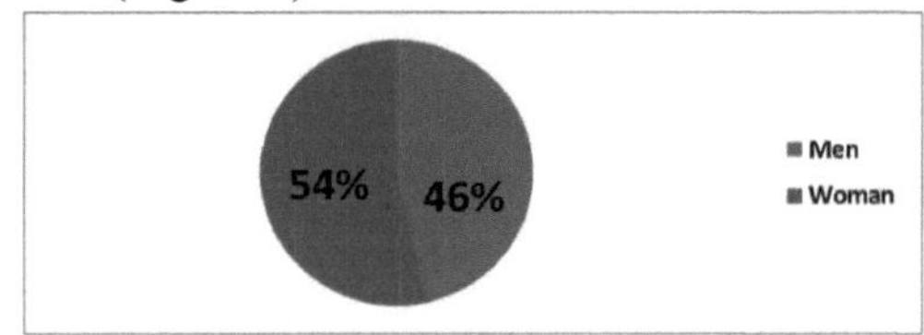

Figure 1: Breakdown of staff by gender

2. Breakdown of staff by age :

According to our results, almost half of the population was in the over 40 (46%) (Figure 2).

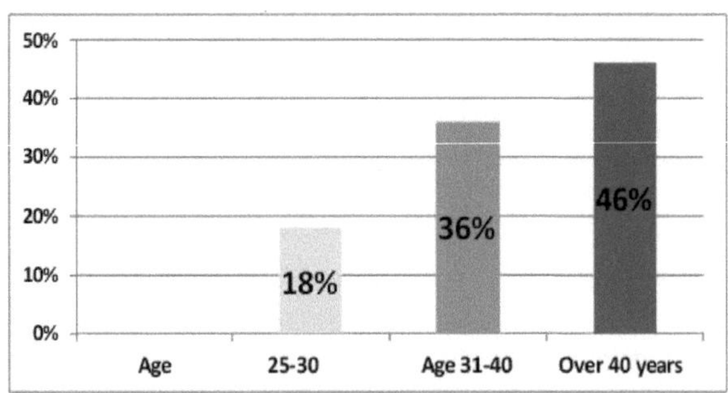

Figure 2: Breakdown of staff by age

3. Breakdown of staff by seniority of work :

The majority of nurses questioned (47%) had been working for more than 10 years (Figure 3).

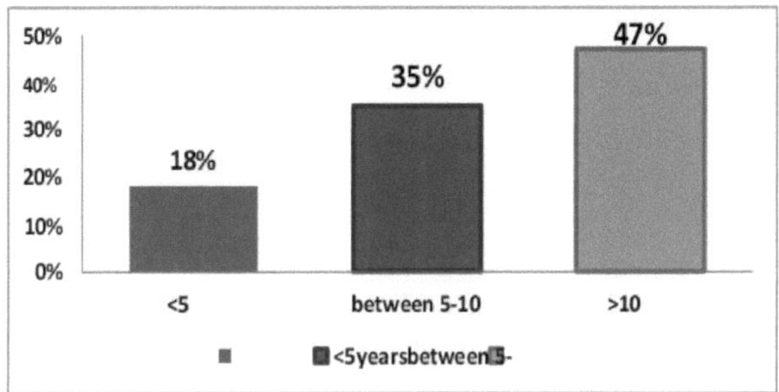

Figure 3: Breakdown of staff by length of service

4. Breakdown of staff by the department hospital :

We found that half of the staff questioned (50%) worked in the emergency department (Figure 4).

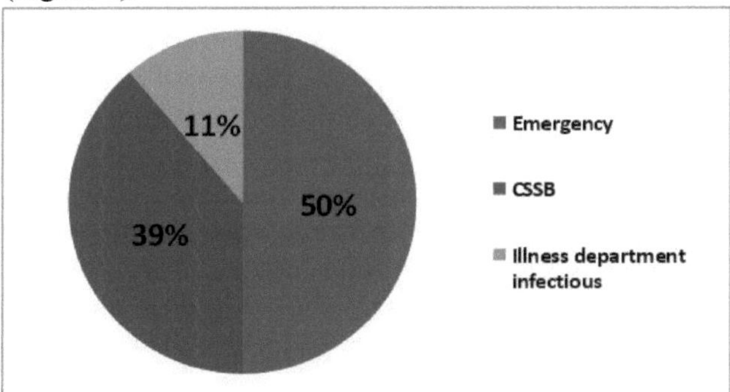

Figure 4: Breakdown of staff by hospital department

B. Study of nurses' knowledge of rabies :

1. Breakdown of staff according to participation in previous training concerning the national rabies control programme :

In our study, 80% of the staff questioned had not received training in the national rabies control programme (Figure 5).

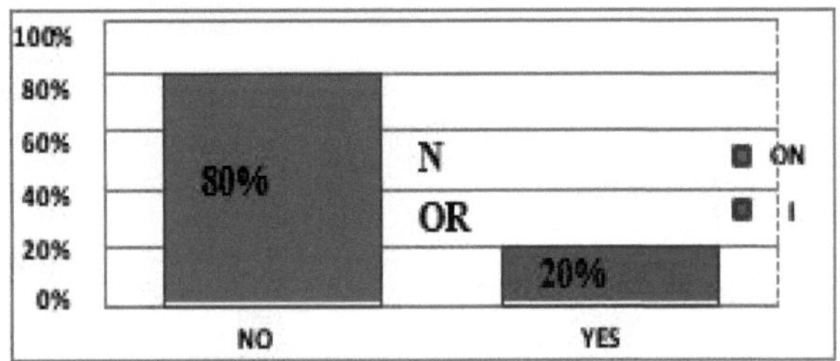

Figure 5: Breakdown of staff by participation in previous training relating to the national programme to combat rabies

In our study, half of the staff questioned (50%) had received training on the national rabies control programme in the EMS department (Figure 6).

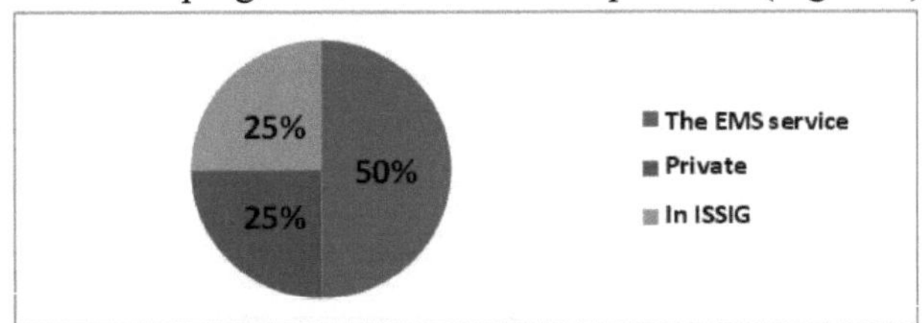

Figure 6: Distribution of staff by training centre for the national rabies control programme

2. Distribution of staff according to responsibility of choice of rabies control protocol:

The majority of staff (70%) replied that the choice of rabies control protocol is a purely medical responsibility (Figure 7).

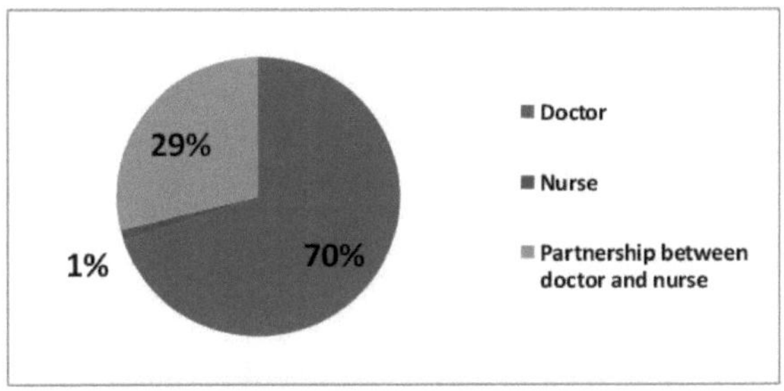

Figure 7: Breakdown of staff by responsibility for protocol choice

3. Breakdown of nurses by type of care case of human rabies :

Most staff (86%) had not previously dealt with a case of human rabies (Figure 8).

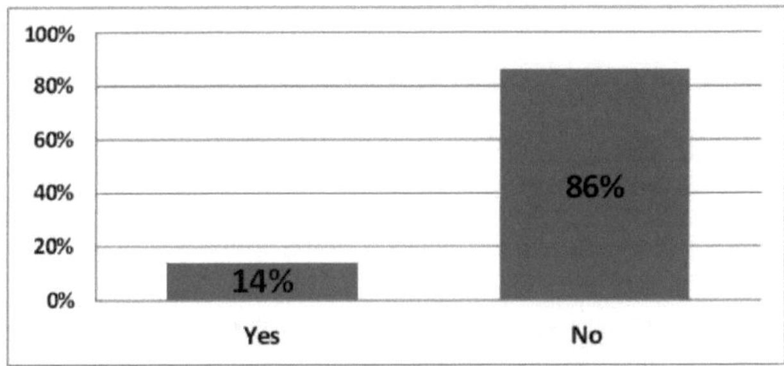

Figure 8: Distribution of staff according to previous treatment of a case of human rabies

C. Study of the degree of implementation of a rabies control protocol :

1. Distribution of staff according to the presence of a rabies control protocol poster in the health facility:

From these results, we noted that 68% of the nurses questioned had a rabies control protocol poster in their health establishment (Figure 9).

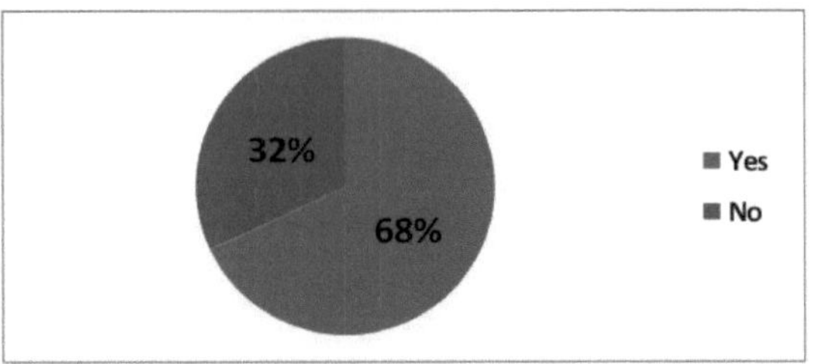

Figure 9: Breakdown of staff by presence a rabies control protocol poster in their health facility

In the absence of this poster, the rest of the participants mentioned the following ways of dealing with the situation (Table 1):

Table 1: Distribution of staff according to the action to be taken in the absence of a rabies control protocol poster in the health facility

What to do	Workforce	Percentage
Contact the doctor manager	24	83%
By memorising the protocol	3	10%
Search for the protocol on social networks	2	7%
Total	29	100%

2. Distribution of staff according to the availability of the resources needed to apply the rabies control protocol :

Most health facilities (60%) had the health resources they needed to apply the rabies control protocol correctly (Figure 10).

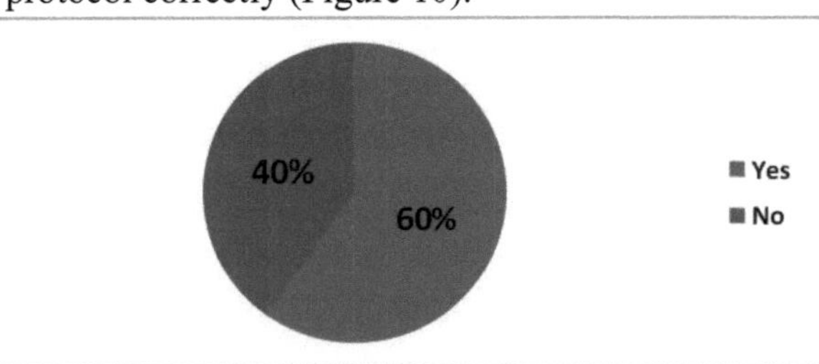

Figure 10: Distribution of staff according to availability of resources needed to apply rabies control protocols

However, a sizeable percentage (40%) had identified the resources that were lacking (Table 2):

Table 2: Breakdown of staff by lack of resources

	Workforce	Percentage
Asepsis equipment	20	62.5%
Anti-rabies serum	8	25%
Tap water	4	12.5%
Total	32	100%

3. Distribution of staff according to degree of compliance with rabies control protocol :

The majority of staff (34%) had an average level of compliance with rabies control protocols (around 50%) (Figure 11).

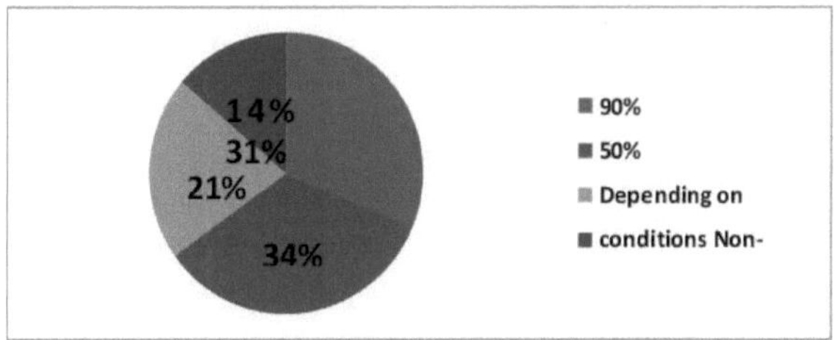

Figure 11: Breakdown of staff by degree of compliance with rabies control protocol

4. Breakdown of staff by obstacles encountered when carrying out rabies control protocols:

Most of the staff questioned (44%) said that their workload was a major obstacle to the acceptable application of the rabies control protocol, despite the presence of the necessary resources (Figure 12).

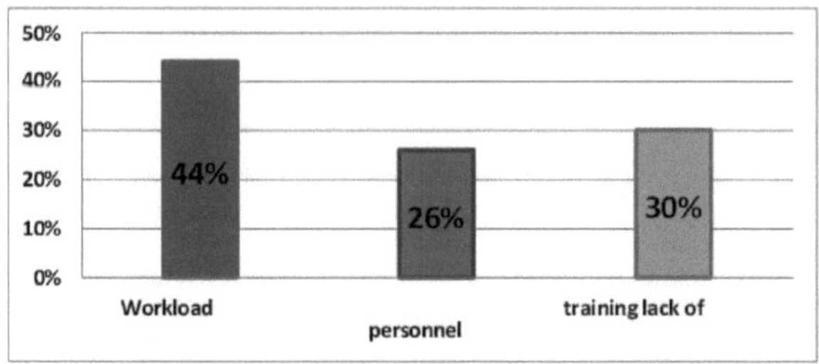

Figure 12: Breakdown of staff by obstacles encountered when carrying out rabies control protocols

5. Distribution of staff according to the first-line action to be taken in the event of an animal bite :

According to the nurses surveyed, "administering rabies serum" was the first thing to be done when faced with a patient bitten by an animal (36%) (Figure 13).

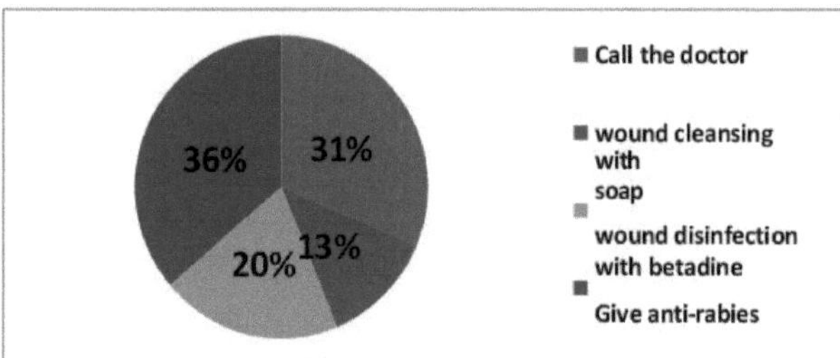

Figure 13: Distribution of staff according to the first action to be taken in the event of an animal bite

6. Distribution of staff according to whether wound cleansing is performed as a first-line treatment.

Of the 80 staff included in our study, we found that only 32% had washed the wound as a first-line treatment after the bite (Figure 14).

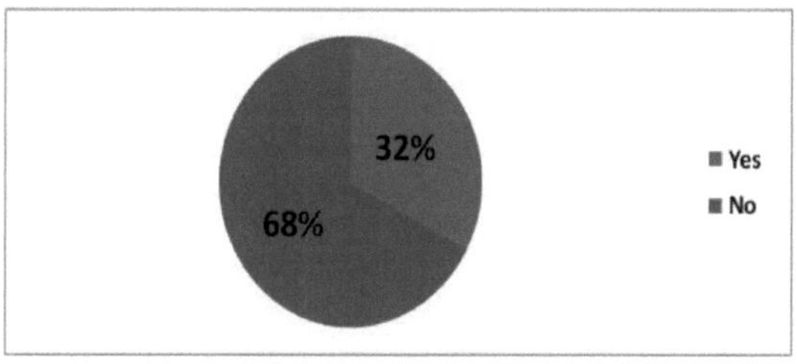

Figure 14: Distribution of staff according to whether wound cleansing was performed as a first-line treatment

Washing times differed from one employee to another (Table 3):

Table 3: Breakdown of staff by duration of wound cleansing

Washing time	Workforce	Percentage
Less than 2 minutes	20	77%
Between 5 and 10 minutes	4	15%
15 minutes	2	8%
Total	26	100%

7. Breakdown of personnel according to test performance of Besredka before infiltration:

We found that the majority of nurses (74%) did not do theBesredka before infiltration (Figure 15). They define the Besredka test as "a test to be carried out before infiltration to detect allergy to rabies serum".

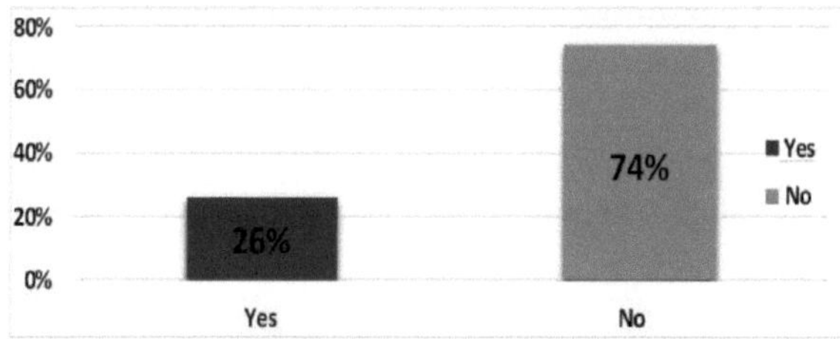

Figure 15: Distribution of personnel according to performance of Besredka test prior to infiltration

8. Breakdown of staff by type of care of a patient allergic to rabies serum:

Most staff (38%) replied that in the event of an allergy to rabies serum, the patient should be admitted to the intensive care unit and the wound infiltrated (Figure 16).

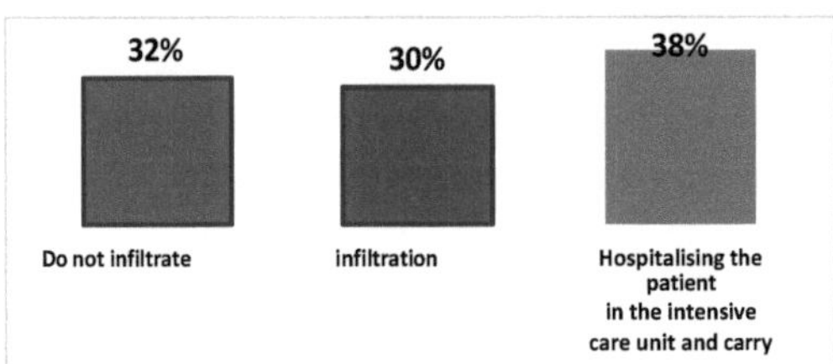

Figure 16: Distribution of staff according to what to do if a patient is allergic to rabies serum

9. Breakdown of staff by the site of infiltration of anti-rabies serum :

The highest percentage of nurses (48%) replied that infiltration is around the wound and intramuscularly (Figure 17).

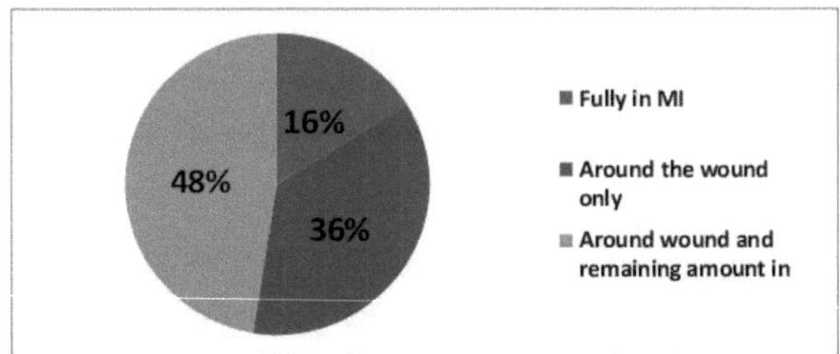

Figure 17: Breakdown of personnel by infiltration site

10. Distribution of personnel according to the application of infiltration in the case of a bite in a sensitive or richly innervated region:

Most nurses (76%) replied that they did not carry out an infiltration in the case of a bite in a sensitive or richly innervated area (Figure 18).

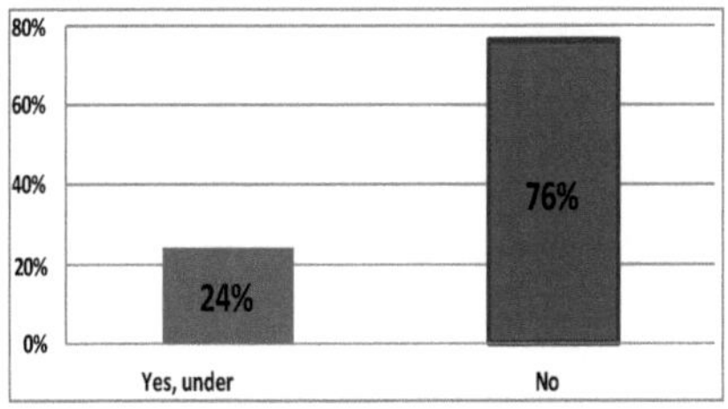

Figure 18: Distribution of personnel according to the application of infiltration in the case of a bite in a sensitive or richly innervated area

11. Distribution of personnel according to suture practice in the event of a major wound :

The majority of staff questioned (61%) replied that they did not suture large wounds (Figure 19).

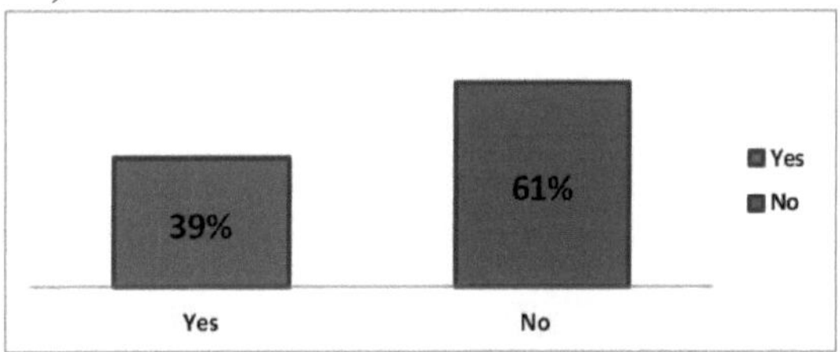

Figure 19: Breakdown of staff by suturing technique for major wounds

The staff interviewed defined the situations in which suturing is possible (Table 4)

Table 4: Distribution of personnel according to possible suture situations

	Workforce	Percentage
24 hours after the bite	29	59%
Reconciliation points if wound larger than 7 cm	20	41%
Total	49	100%

D. Study of prevention measures :

1. Breakdown of staff by patient education :

We concluded that the majority of staff (66%) were unaware of the importance of patient education (Figure 20).

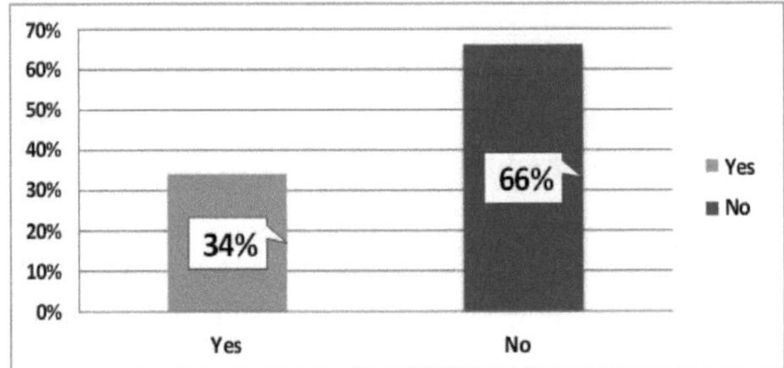

Figure 20: Distribution of staff according to patient education

The educational themes mentioned by the staff were :
*Immediate wound cleansing after an animal bite
*Importance of arriving quickly to vaccinate
*Follow the appropriate vaccination schedule.

2. Distribution of staff according to the action to be taken in the event of delayed vaccination by patients:

In our survey, 62% of staff responded with "Nothing to do, it's not my job". In this way, it is possible to avoid "liability" in the event of delayed vaccination by patients (Figure 21).

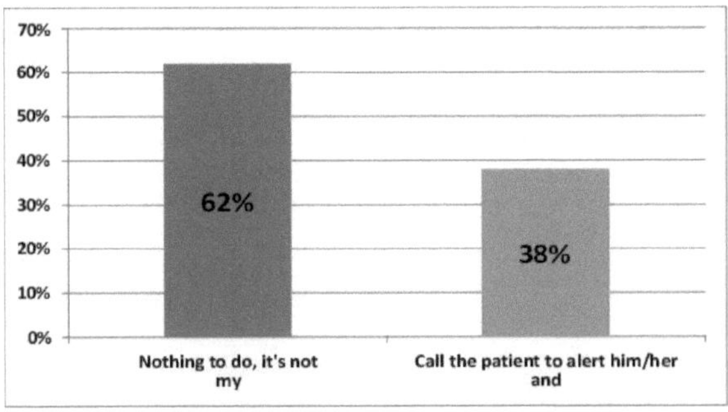

Figure 21: Distribution of staff by action to be taken in the event of delayed vaccination by patients

IV. ANALYSIS OF QUESTIONNAIRE RESULTS FROM THE VICTIM POPULATION

During our study period, 75 participants who had been bitten by an animal were included.

1. Socio-demographic data :

1.1. Breakdown of victims by age :

In our target population, the 30-35 age group was the most common (41%) (Table 5).

Table 5: Breakdown of victims by age

Tranche age	Workforce	Percentage (%)
[18-30[	29	39
[30-35[	31	41
35 and over	15	20
Total	75	100

1.2. Breakdown of victims by gender :

The majority of patients interviewed were male (64%), with a sex ratio (M/F) of 2.84 (Figure 22).

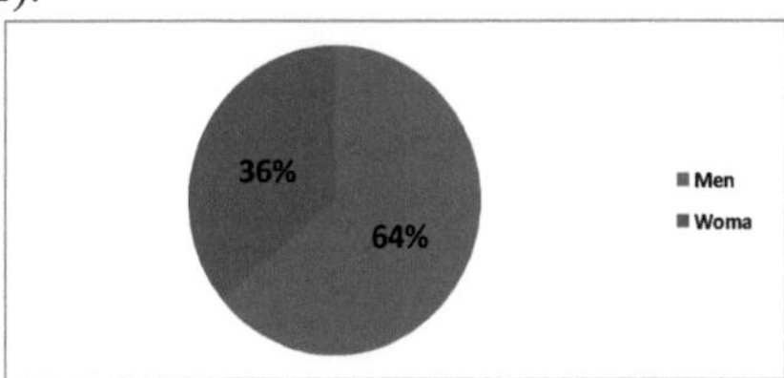

Figure 22: Breakdown of victims by gender

1.3. Breakdown of the victme population by geographical origin :

Most of the participants were from urban areas (60%) (Figure23).

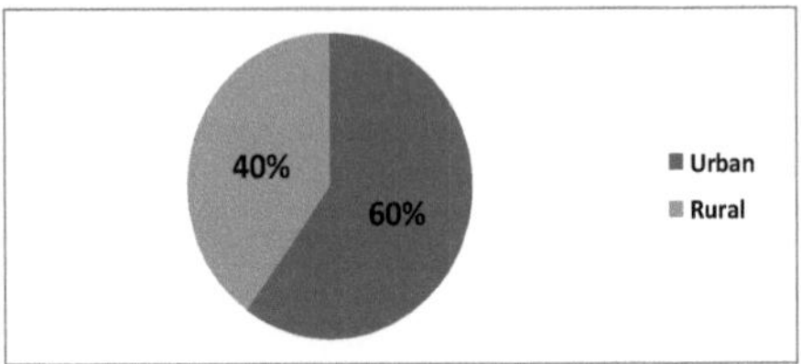

Figure 23: Breakdown of victims by geographical origin

1.4. Breakdown of the victme population by level of instruction :

The majority of respondents had no more than primary education (60%) (Figure24).

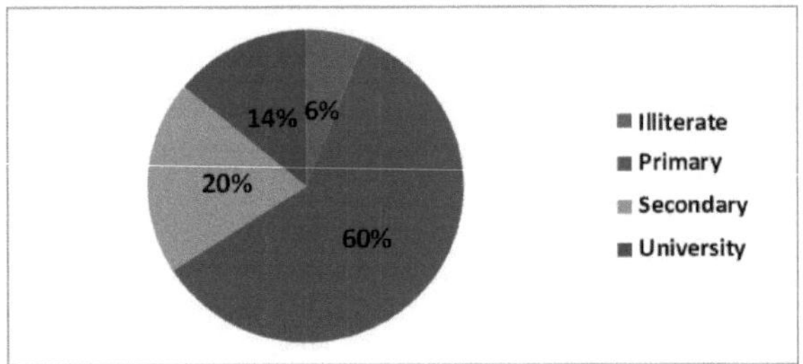

Figure 24: Breakdown of victims by level of education

1.5. Breakdown of the victme population by profession :

Of the respondents, 42% were professionally active (Figure 25). Also, 26% of this category were self-employed (Table 6):

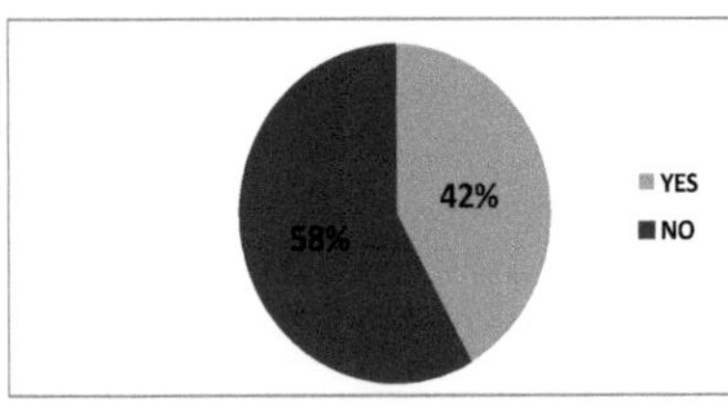

Figure 25: Breakdown of victims by occupation Table6: Breakdown of victims by occupation

Profession	Workforce	Percentage
Senior executive	5	19%
Senior executive	1	4%
Middle management	12	44%
Worker	2	7%
Liberal profession	7	26%
Total	27	100%

1.6. Breakdown of the Victorian population by socio-economic level :

The majority of patients of study (55%) had an average socio-economic level (Figure 26).

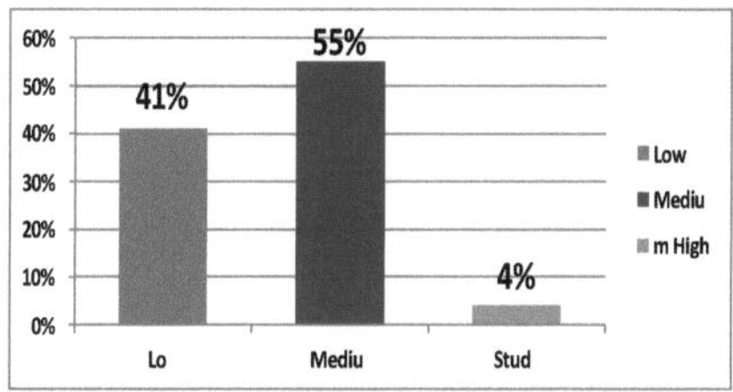

Figure 26: Breakdown of victims by socio-economic level

2. Study of the knowledge of the victim population about animal bites:

2.1. Distribution of the Victorian population according to awareness of the fatal risk of rabies :

Based on these results, we found that the majority of the victim population (73%) thought that rabies is a fatal disease (Figure27).

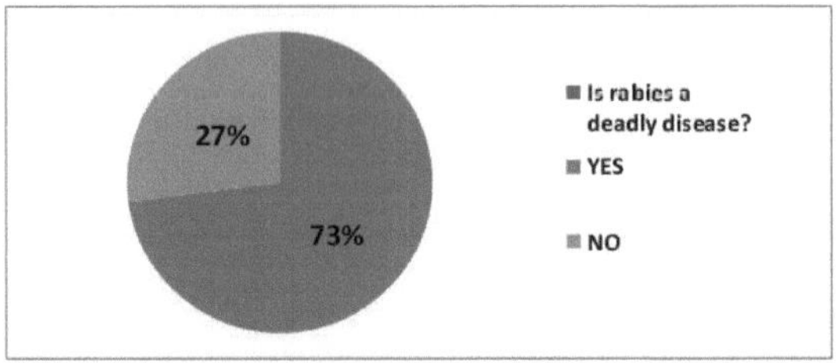

Figure 27: Distribution of the victim population according to awareness of the fatal risk of rabies

2.2. Distribution of victims according to knowledge of the animal rage transmitter

According to these results, the majority of participants (60%) thought that rabies can only be transmitted by dogs (Figure 28).

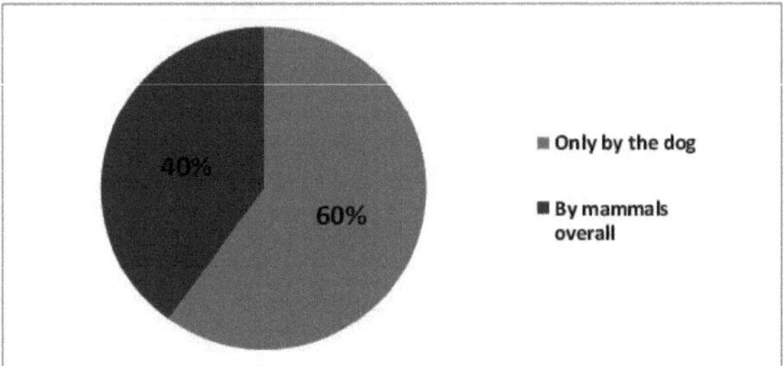

Figure 28: Breakdown of the victim population according to knowledge of the animal responsible for rabies transmission

2.3. Distribution of the Victorian population according to human-to-human transmission of rabies :

We found that the majority of the victim population (83%) agreed with the possibility of human-to-human transmission of rabies (Figure 29).

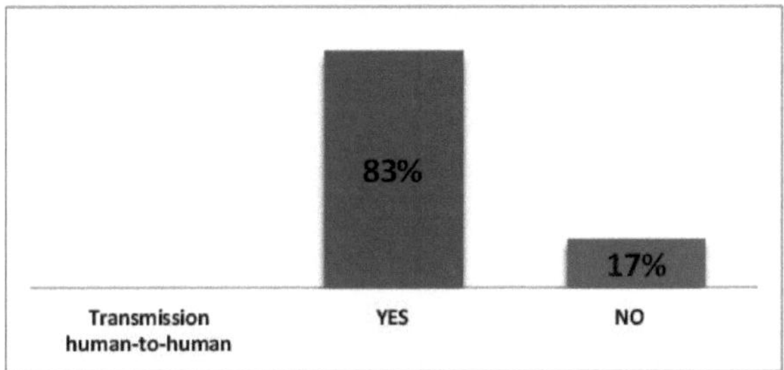

Figure 29: Distribution of the victim population according to knowledge of human-to-human transmission of rabies

2.4 Distribution of the Victorian population according to the possibility of contracting rabies from an object licked by a rabid animal:

More than half (61%) agreed with the possibility of catching rabies during a contact with an object licked by a rabid animal (Figure30).

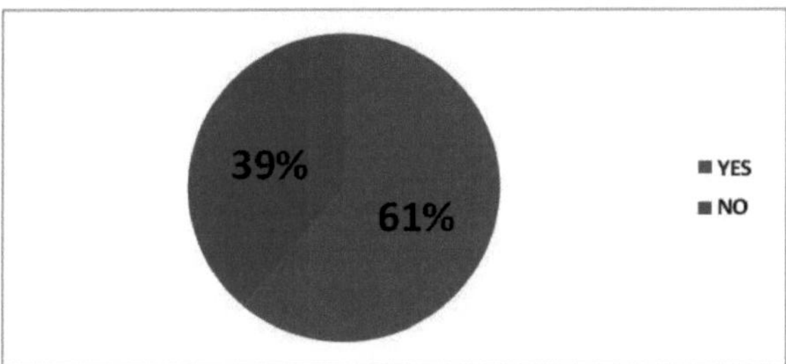

Figure 30: Breakdown of the victim population according to the possibility of contracting rabies from an object licked by a rabid animal

2.5 Breakdown of the Victorian population according to awareness of signs suggestive of rabies :

In our study, 25% of participants voted for all the proposals given that evoked rabies (Figure31).

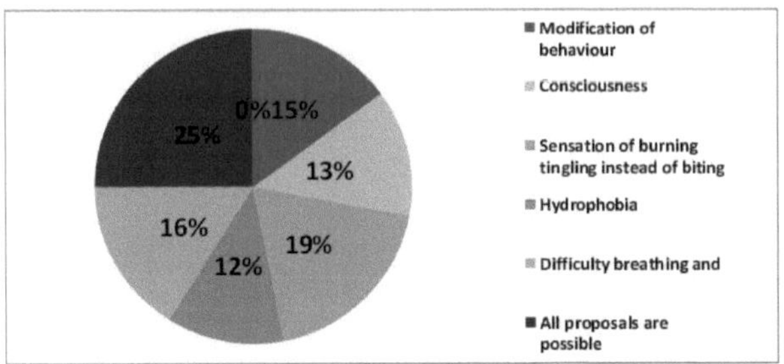

Figure 31: Distribution of the victim population according to choice of signs of human rabies

2.6 Breakdown of the Victorian population according to the first-line response to a bite from a suspected rabid animal :

Of the 75 participants, 55% would go to the nearest health centre if they were bitten by a suspect animal (Figure 32).

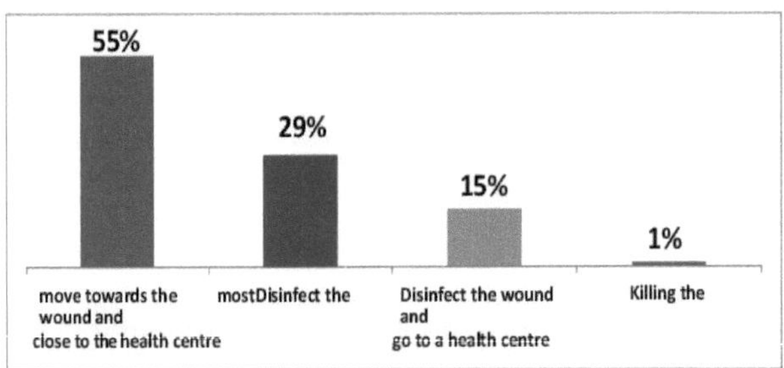

Figure 32: Distribution of participants according to first-line response to a bite from a suspected rabid animal

2.7 The first point of contact in the event of an animal bite:

Most participants (69%) would go to the emergency department in the event of an animal bite (Figure 33).

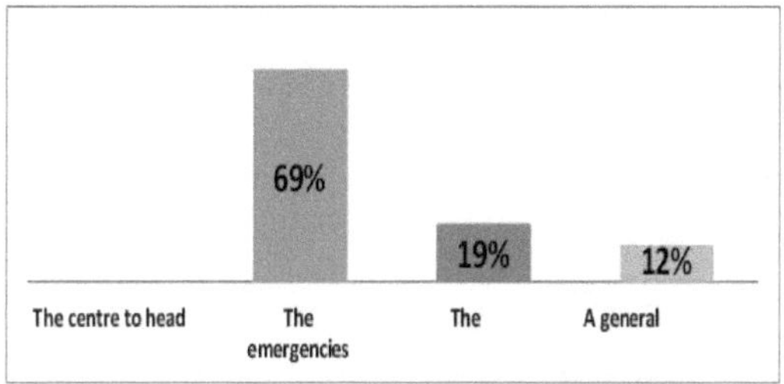

Figure 33: Distribution of participants according to the first centre to go to in the event of an animal bite

2.8 Breakdown of the victme population by time of arrival for rabies vaccination :

54% of participants arrived for vaccination on the same day (D0) after the bite (Figure 34).

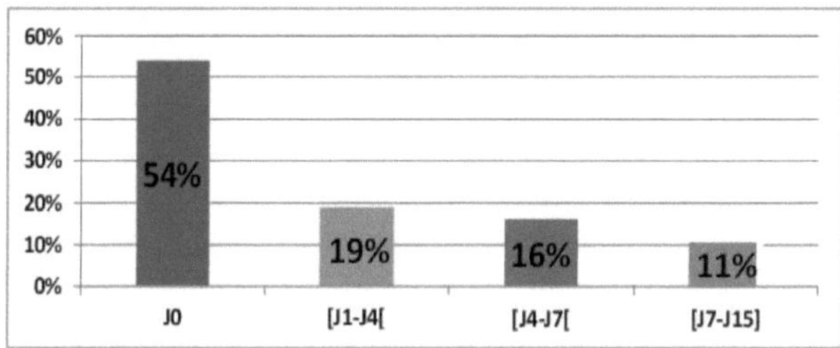

Figure 34: Distribution of participants according to arrival time for rabies vaccination

2.9 Distribution of the victme population according to the performance of post-bite wound cleansing :

We found that 56% of participants did not wash the wound immediately after a bite (Figure 35).

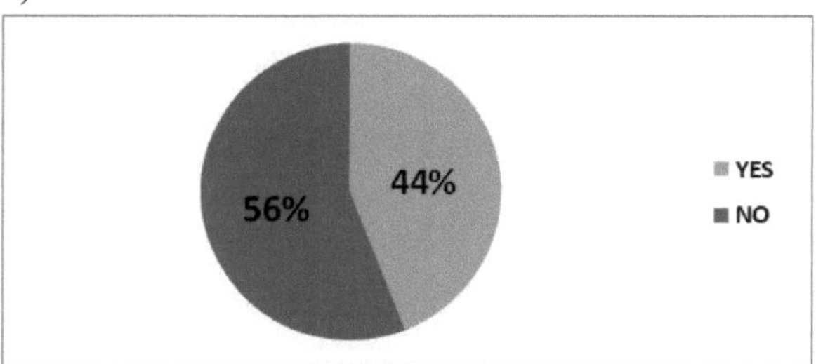

Figure 35: Distribution of participants according to how they performed wound cleansing

The cleansing product differed from one participant to another. The most commonly used product was water with Marseille soap (52%) (Figure 36).

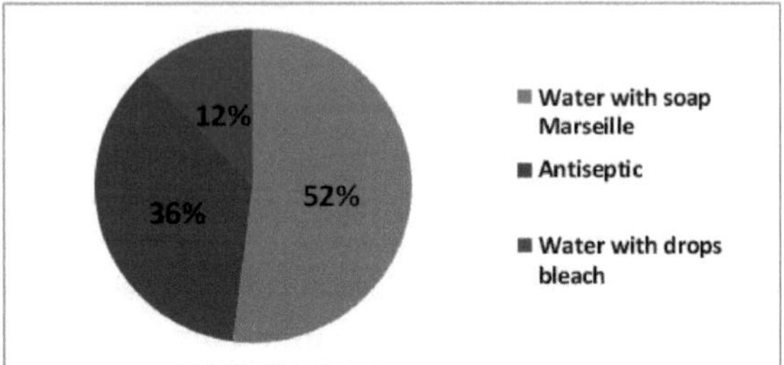

Figure 36: Distribution of participants according to the washing product used

According to our results, the duration of washing was not the same for all participants: From this graph, we can see that more than half (52%) washed their car at least once a week.for a maximum of 2 minutes (Figure37).

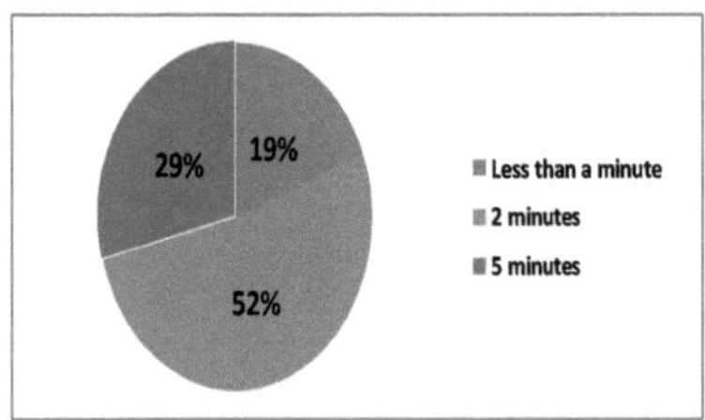

Figure 37: Distribution of participants according to duration of wound cleansing

2.10Breakdown of the victme population according to booster vaccination schedule :

We found that the highest percentage (58%) was for participants who followed the booster vaccination schedule (Figure 38).

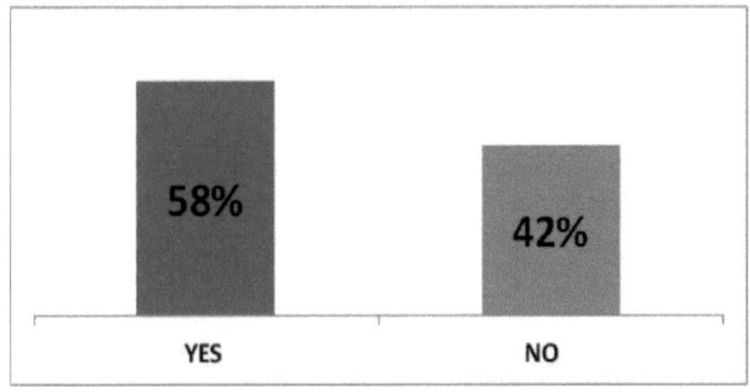

Figure 38: Distribution of participants according to follow-up of booster vaccinations according to the vaccination schedule

The remaining participants (42%) gave the following reasons for not following up: irresponsibility (41%), lack of transport (34%) and workload (25%) (Figure 39).

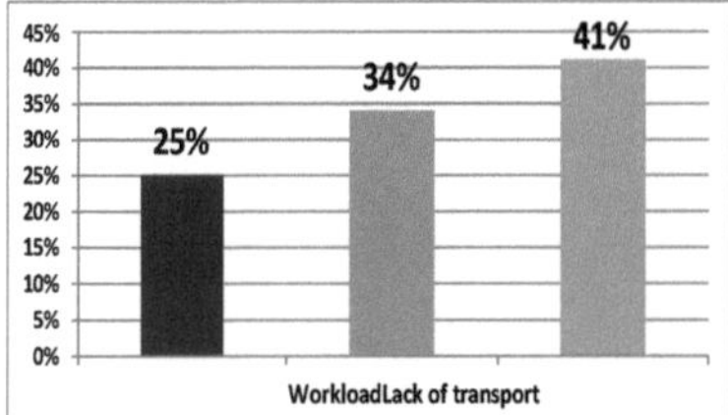

Figure 39: Breakdown of participants by reason for not attending booster vaccinations

2.11 Breakdown of the Victorian population according to the number o f veterinary visits requested in cases of suspected rabies :

We found that 53% of victims had been visited by vets in the event of suspected animal rabies (Figure 40).

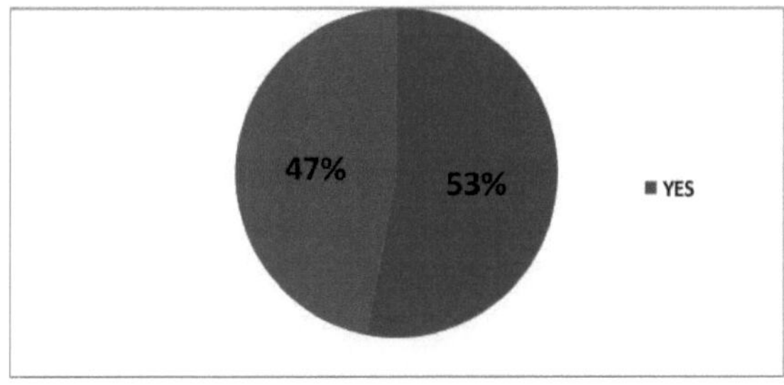

Figure 40: Distribution of participants according to veterinary visits carried out in cases of suspected rabies

2.12 Breakdown of the victme population according to knowledge of mandatory reporting of rabies :

We found that the majority (88%) voted in favour of compulsory declaration in cases of rabies (Figure 41).

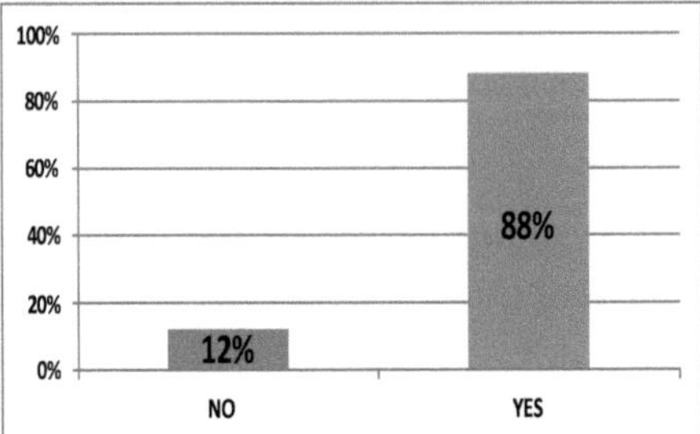

Figure 41: Distribution of participants according to awareness of the obligation to report cases of rabies

V. GENERAL INFORMATION ON RABIES

1. Definition :

Rabies is an anthropozoonosis that can affect all warm-blooded animals, which are both reservoirs and vectors of the rabies virus. Rabies is a fatal encephalomyelitis whose aetiological agents are grouped within the Lyssavirus genus [4]. After a long incubation period, the disease is characterised by encephalomyelitis, which is generally fatal and is usually accompanied by signs of excitation, aggression or paralysis. Rabies is a notifiable disease [5].

2. Symptoms

Symptomatology remains highly artificial in the various susceptible species because of the two extreme forms (furious and paralytic), variations and combinations of which are conceivable [6].

2.1. In dogs :

There are two possible types of rabies in dogs:

✓ **Furious rabies:** lasts 1 to 2 months and then evolves in 3 phases:

-Prodromal phase: the first signs of rabies are simple changes in the animal's habits. The dog is anxious and less obedient. This phase lasts 24 hours.

- **State phase:** there is a simultaneous or successive appearance of psychological, aggressive and nervous signs. The dog is agitated and worried, then suddenly calms down and lies down; the dog's voice changes. It lets out a muffled, hoarse howl, with two tones that represent the "rabid cry"; the animal then becomes furious and aggressive, biting everything in sight. This aggressiveness is highlighted by the sign of the stick. The dog flees straight ahead, its eyes haggard, in a state of confusion. psychomotor skills and bites if it is prevented from escaping. The pharynx is paralysed

causing difficulty swallowing and drooling.

- **Terminal phase:** Ascending paralysis begins in the posterior train and leads to rapid death in 4 or 5 days. [7].

•**Paralytic or mute rabies:** this is characterised by the appearance of an infection caused by paralysis. With a dropped jaw, the dog cannot bite, eat, drink or cry out. This silent form is rare and develops over 4 days [8].

2.2. In humans :

Rabies in humans is presented as acute meningoencephalitis (Aubry et al., 2001)[6]. The incubation period depends on the site of the bite. In 85% of cases, it lasts between 35 and 90 days. The prodromal stages of the disease last 2 to 4 days. The symptoms are essentially sensory: pain in the bitten area, tingling, profound sadness, crying spells for no reason, seeking isolation. The temperature may rise by 1 to 3 degrees. During the state period, character disorders become more pronounced. The patient, extremely distressed, is prey to hallucinations and irradiated pain. The temperature can rapidly reach 41-42°C. Symptoms come in a variety of forms:

❖ **The spastic form**, characterised by violent contractures and tremors. Sensory stimuli such as light, sound or touch trigger very painful spasms, particularly of the larynx, altering the voice and making swallowing painful. Hydrophobia is a very common symptom. characteristic of humans. Towards the end, bulbar disorders appear. The patient's intelligence remains intact until the final coma. Death occurs in 2 to 10 days.

❖ **The paralytic form** may begin with monoplegia, paraplegia or paralysis. take on the appearance of ascending paralysis. In this form, the diagnosis is made particularly difficult when the notion of a bite is lacking, and in the case of regions where there is little or no rabies. Death occurs later through respiratory paralysis when the bulbar region is affected.

❖ **The dementia form** is characterised by exacerbated aggressiveness with fits of raving madness, rapidly progressing to coma and death [9].

1.3 Treatment :

In animals, no treatment for rabies has been declared [10], but in humans, various therapies have been tried, such as the use of anti-rabies serums after exposure, which is a specific treatment, and also the injection of interferons, which is non-specific. However, to date, clinically declared rabies is always fatal [11]. For local treatment of wounds where there is a risk of infection, first aid consists of eliminating the rabies virus at the site of infection by chemical or physical means. Immediate cleaning with soap and water, followed by rinsing with water, is necessary. Then apply either 40-70% alcohol, tincture of iodine or an iodine solution, which must be supplemented by treatment under medical supervision in accordance with the protocol defined by the WHO with the mixed sero-vaccine treatment, which must be rigorously followed by the attending physician. The protocol comprises 4 injections and 2 subcutaneous booster doses at 30 and 90 days of the vaccine after administration of the anti-rabies serum immediately after the bite, so there is a local treatment, anti-rabies serotherapy and anti-rabies vaccination.

❖ **Local treatment of lesions :**

► Immediately wash the seat thoroughly with plenty of water. the exhibition.

► Apply a lethal product to the rabies virus.

► Do not suture the wound immediately.

❖ **Rabies serotherapy :**

► Before any administration of a serum anti-rabies serum heterologous serum,it is A skin sensitivity test using the Besredka method is recommended.

► Where indicated, rabies serum should be used topically at the following dosage dose of 40 IU per kg of body weight.

❖ **Rabies vaccination** :

• The vaccine must be reconstituted with one ampoule of solvent per dose. Once reconstituted, the vaccine must be used immediately.

• Route of administration: the vaccine must be administered intramuscularly, unless otherwise stated:

► In adults: in the deltoid muscle.

► In children under 4: in the quadriceps.

► Exceptionally in case of contraindication from the intramuscular route, the subcutaneous route may be used.

• Treatments are classified into four types of protocol called: **A1, A2, B1** and **B2 (Figure 42)**.

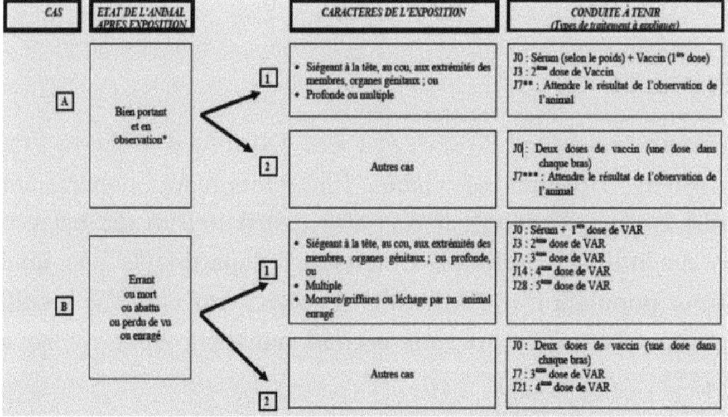

Figure 42: Rabies control protocol

VI. STUDY OF NURSING KNOWLEDGE ON RABIES

1.Socio-demographic data :

1.1 Sex :

During the study period, 80 staff were included. The sex ratio was 0.6, indicating a predominance of women (54% women). A survey carried out in Indonesia on a sample of 153 nurses also showed a predominance of women, with a sex ratio of 0.3, which is consistent with our study [12]. In addition, the results of a survey carried out in Djaména involving 86 healthcare professionals showed that most of them were men (64.8%) [13].

1.2. Age :

During our survey, we noted a predominance of people aged over 40 (46%). This is similar to the results found in the same study in Djaména (67% between 40 and 50 years of age, with an average age of 47 ± 10.07 years) [13]. In a similar study carried out in Morocco, they found that the average age of participants was 42 ± 13 years (with extremes ranging from 27 to 53 years). Two-thirds (n = 107; 65%) of the nurses were in the 20-49 age group. [14].

1.3 Seniority :

In terms of length of service, the majority of staff had more than 10 years' service (47%), while the results of a survey carried out in Morocco showed that more than two-thirds of the 4168 staff had more than ten years' service (average length of service = 12.6 ± 8.3 years) [14].

1.4 Services :

Our questionnaire concerned 80 staff and was distributed to the two departments of the University Hospital of Gabès (the emergency department and the infectious diseases department); it was also distributed to the basic health care centres and the military hospital. Emergency departments accounted for the majority of our population (50%), which is consistent with the results found in Bali, Indonesia, where 77% of staff carried out their work in the emergency department [12].

2. Study of nurses' knowledge about rabies and the extent to which the rabies control protocol has been implemented:

1. Study of nurses' knowledge of rabies

1.1 Rabies training :

The classification of staff according to participation in previous training concerning the national rabies control programme showed that (80%) of the staff questioned had not undergone training. This may explain the failures in the management of cases at risk of contracting human rabies that have been reported in Tunisia, and the deaths of some cases. French surveys have shown that 73% of nurses had received training in rabies risk management [15].

c:> **Rabies is a national programme, and it is essential that the staff involved in this protocol take part in ongoing training to keep up to date with any changes to the protocol, as well as new developments in care and prevention to improve the results.**

1.2 The choice of protocol :

70% of staff said that the choice of protocol was a joint responsibility between the doctor and the nurse. Only 1% of participants said that the nurse was responsible for choosing the rabies protocol.

c:> **The choice of protocol is the responsibility of the doctor, but may be in collaboration with the nurse, since the 1er contact with the victim is with the nurse.**

2. Study the degree of execution of the rabies protocol :

2.1 The protocol poster :

Concerning the distribution of staff according to the presence of a poster of the rabies protocol in their health establishment, we noted that the majority of nurses questioned (68%) had a poster of the protocol in the treatment rooms of their departments, while the rest of the nurses (32%) stated that there were no posters of the protocol. This presents a problem for good practice and correct execution of the protocol. In the absence of the posters, nurses mentioned the alternative of contacting the doctor in charge to manage the situation (83%). In Toronto, the Minister of Health published the Ontario Public Health Standards: Requirements for Programs, Services and Accountability (the Standards) under section 7 of the Health Protection and Promotion Act (HPPA) to specify the importance of the presence of rabies protocol posters in health services. Indeed, the presence of the poster is mandatory in the departments [16]. In a similar study carried out in Saudi Arabia, 87% of staff stated that rabies control protocol posters and awareness posters were present in emergency departments and infectious diseases departments [17].

c:> **It is necessary for the protocol poster to be displayed on the premises of to facilitate implementation, improve care and avoid complications.**

2.2. Health averages :

In our study, the majority of participants (60%) had the necessary health resources to apply the rabies protocol. The survey carried out by the Agence National de Sécurité des Médicaments et des Produits de Sante (National Agency for the Safety of Medicines and Health Products) in Saint Denis, France, reported results similar to our own (57%): they had the necessary health resources to apply the rabies control protocol [18].However, a sizeable percentage (40%) had identified a lack of resources, essentially a lack of aseptic equipment (soap, alcohol, Betadine), bearing in mind that asepsis and washing reduce the possibility of catching rabies by 40%, and 25% mentioned a lack of anti-rabies serum, which is considered to be one of the most important tools for preventing rabies contamination.

2.3. The degree of protocol execution :

The distribution of staff according to the degree of compliance with the rabies control protocol showed that the majority of staff (34%) had a degree of compliance with this protocol of around 50%; and that a sizeable percentage (14%) of participants did not comply correctly with the protocol. These results were not consistent with those found in Djaména, where 77% of staff complied with the rabies control protocol to the order of 90% [13].

2.4. The first line of defence is :

With regard to the distribution of staff according to the first-line action to be taken in the event of an animal bite, we noted that the heading "give anti-rabies serum" was the most frequently chosen (36%). Only 13% of staff washed the wound with soap and water. We also found that (20%) of the nurses disinfected the wound with Betadine, but this was not enough. In a similar study carried out in the emergency department in Canada, it was found that, as soon as victims of animal bites arrived, the first things to be done were: i) to wash the wounds in 70% of cases, ii) to do nothing in 20% and iii) to apply traditional care such as wound disinfection (with Betadine, alcohol, etc.). ...)in 7.4% of cases [19].

c:> **Washing the wound with soap and water is the first step to take in the event of an animal bite (1[er]).**

2.5. Washing time :

Among the 80 staff included in our study, we noted that only (32%) washed the wound as a first line of defence after the bite, and we noted that the duration of washing differed from one staff member to another. We noted that the majority (60%) completed washing in less than 2 minutes, and only 10% of respondents took 15 minutes to wash the wound. In a Canadian study, 67% of staff washed for between 7 and 15 minutes, which is not consistent with our results [19].

2.6. The Besredka test :

The Besredka test is a pre-infiltration test to detect allergy to rabies serum. In our study, we found that the majority of nurses (74%) did not carry out this test before infiltration. This can cause a number of anaphylactic problems and may be the cause of death in some subjects who have developed allergies to rabies serum. An Indian study reported that 66% of nurses did not perform the Besredka test prior to rabies serum infiltration [20].

:> **This test is considered a medico-legal responsibility.**

With regard to what to do when faced with a patient allergic to rabies serum, we noted that most staff (38%) replied that the patient should be admitted to the intensive care unit and the wound infiltrated. The results of a study carried out in India showed similar results, with 47% of staff stating that it was necessary to admit the patient to the intensive care unit and infiltrate the wound with a metrostatic monitor, given the risk of anaphylactic shock [21].

c:> **If a patient has an allergy to anti-rabies serum, the vaccination and hospitalise him in the intensive care unit for infiltration and monitor its condition regularly.**

2.7. The vaccination route :

Infiltration should be done around the wound and intramuscularly. In our study, the highest percentage of nurses (48%) answered that infiltration is done around the wound and intramuscularly. The results of a survey carried out in India were similar and showed that according to 44% of nurses, infiltration is done around the wound and the rest is done intramuscularly [21].

The vaccine dose, which is the same for both adults and children, must be administered intramuscularly (IM):

- **In adults: in the deltoid muscle (upper third of the arm at the middle of the deltoid V)**

- **In children under 4 years of age: the entire dose is injected into the quadriceps (middle third of the outer anterolateral surface of the thigh). In exceptional cases where the I.M. route is contraindicated (subjects on anticoagulants, haemophiliacs, etc.), the subcutaneous route (s/c) may be used: in the lower third of the posterior aspect of the forearm, compressing the injection site for 5 minutes.**

c:> **Infiltration should be given around the wound and the rest intramuscularly.**

Concerning the distribution of personnel according to the application of the infiltration in the event of a bite in a sensitive or richly innervated region, our results showed that most nurses (76%) answered not to apply the infiltration in the event of a bite in a sensitive or richly innervated region.

2.8. The suture :

According to our study, 61% of the staff questioned replied that they did not suture a large wound. The results of an Indian study showed that 78% of staff sutured after the bite, which is not consistent with our results [20].
Do not suture the wound immediately. However, if suturing is unavoidable, it should only be carried out several hours after the local administration of rabies immunoglobulin, using a very limited number of stitches.

.3 Study of prevention measures :

Correct implementation of the protocol is the primary means of preventing human rabies. Also, in order to limit the emergence of new cases of rabies, victims need to be properly educated about bites and the first steps to be taken. To achieve this, public awareness and education must be stepped up through the media and awareness campaigns, with the aim of reducing the incidence of human rabies. In our study, the distribution of staff according to patient education showed that the majority of staff (66%) were unaware of the importance of patient education. The education themes mentioned by staff were :

*Washing the wound immediately after an animal bite,

*The importance of arriving promptly for vaccination

*The importance of following the correct vaccination schedule.

3.1 What to do if vaccination is delayed :

Concerning the distribution of staff according to the action to be taken in the event of delayed vaccination by patients, 62% of staff replied "Nothing to do, it's not my responsibility". The second response was "It's our responsibility and we have to declare it and call the patient to start the protocol" in 48% of cases.

c:> **The nurse's responsibility is not just to wash and vaccinate, but also to play a vital role in educating people, raising awareness, monitoring and even evaluating the effectiveness of the treatment. the degree of effectiveness of the treatment and vaccine given. This allows us toimprove care and reduce the associated morbidity and mortality.**

c:> **So we need to reorganise the tasks in the establishments and provide ongoing training for the staff. Also, we must not forget to provide the materials needed to carry out the protocol correctly.**

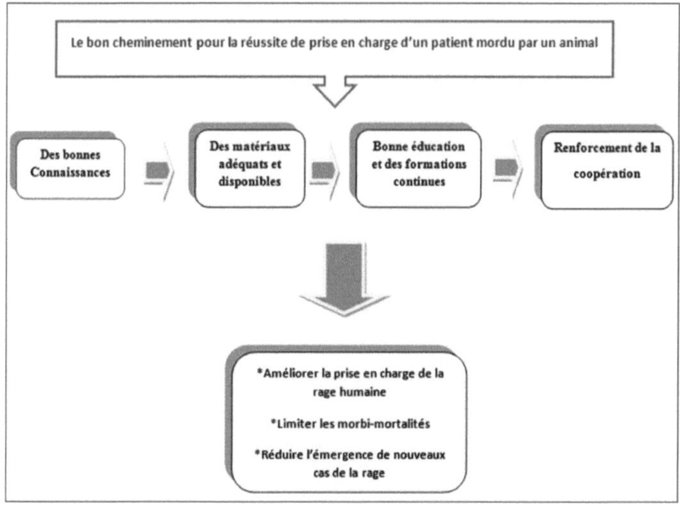

3. Study of rabies-related knowledge in victims of animal bites :

1.Socio-demographic data :

1.1.Sex:

During the study period, 75 patients were included. The sex ratio was

2. 84 in favour of a male predominance (74% men). This predominance was also noted in a study carried out including 1000 victims hospitalised in the city of Bamako (a male predominance of 90% with a sex ratio of 0.9) [22]. In a descriptive study carried out in Bizerte, 64% of the 348 victims who took part in the survey were women. [23].

1.2. Age:

In our study, 41% of respondents were in the 30-35 age group. In a study carried out in the city of Bamako [22], 71% of victims were aged under 30.

1.3. Geographical origin :

According to the results of our study, 60% of the subjects were of urban origin, whereas in the study carried out in the city of Bamako, 86% of the participants were ofrural origin [22].

c:> **We can conclude that geographical origin differs from one study to another another, which may give a further argument that rabies is not limited to one geographical area, despite the difference in living conditions.**

1.4. Level of education :

Concerning the level of education of the population studied, we concluded that 60% of the subjects studied had no more than primary education, and these results are not consistent with the results of a study carried out in the city of Cotonou, where the level of primary education of 259 people constituted only 12.3% of the population [24]. However, in another study carried out in the city of Bamako, the predominance of the primary level was marked and was equal to 72% [22].

c:> **Based on these data, we found that the predominance of level A factor that may explain the difficulties or poor implementation of the rabies control protocol is the fact that there is no primary prevention of rabies in the victim population.**

1.5. Socio-economic level :

According to our results, the majority of the subjects included had an average socioeconomic level (55%) and this predominance was also noted in a study carried out in Bizerte (68.5%) [23].

c:> **Socio-economic status is a key factor in the successful management of bites. In fact, the material aspect is an important pillar of treatment. to complete the rabies care pathway.**

2.Study of rabies awareness among victims of animal bites:

2.1.The fatal risk of rabies:

In our study, we found that (73%) of the subjects included did not think that rabies is a fatal disease. This majority was also found in a survey of 348 participants in Bizerte (87.6%) [23].

c:> **One of the risk factors for mortality caused by rabies and for delays in treatment is unawareness of the seriousness of the disease and the heavy costs involved. consequences and mortality of this disease.**

2.2.The animal that transmits rabies :

In our study, 60% of participants thought that rabies is transmitted solely by dogs. In the Bizerte study, the majority (67.4%) were aware that rabies can be transmitted by species other than dogs [23].

c:> **These results have enabled us to confirm that population ignorance victim of the epidemiology and modes of transmission of rabies represented a major risk to the spread of rabies today.**

2.3.Human-to-human transmission of rabies :

According to our results, we found that the majority of the victim population (83%) thought that there was a possibility of human-to-human transmission of rabies, which is in line with a study carried out in Abidjan, where the majority (61%) of those questioned affirmed the existence of human-to-human transmission of rabies [25].

c:> **According to WHO data, human-to-human transmission by bite or saliva is theoretically possible, but has never been confirmed and no cases have been reported worldwide.**

2.4. Signs of rabies in humans:

With regard to signs suggestive of rabies, in our study we found behavioural disorders (15%) and hydrophobia (12%). In the study carried out in Abidjan, the same signs were described with a percentage of 20% [25].

c:> **This concordance between two different studies on the signs suggestive of rabies in humans has enabled us to confirm an acceptable level of knowledge about the disease under study, which will make it possible to to raise the issue of the disease early on, to ensure that it is treated as quickly as possible.**

2.5. What to do in the first instance following a bite by a animal :

When we studied the first-line response to a bite, we found the following results: referral to a health facility (55%), wound disinfection (29%), wound disinfection and referral to a health centre (15%), kill the animal (1%). In the Cotonou study, the team found the same courses of action but with different percentages: referral to a health facility, disinfection of the wound and referral to a health centre. (84.6%), washing and disinfection of the wound (0.8%), referral to a health facility with wound washing (0.4%), killing the animal (1.9%) [24].

c:> **Despite the fact that the correct course of action was "disinfection of the wound and referral to a health centre", she did not have the highest percentage in different studies. This may explain the shortcomings in management, with a significant possibility of increasing the risk of rabies-related morbidity and mortality.**

2.6. The first place to go if you've been bitten by an animal:

In our study, the results differed from one participant to another regarding the first centre to go to after an animal bite: 69% went to the emergency department, 12% consulted a doctor and 19% went to a basic healthcare centre. Among 89 members surveyed in a study conducted in Bizerte, 47.2% went to hospital, 6.7% consulted a doctor and 41.6% went to a basic healthcare centre [23].

c:> **Based on this comparison, we found that the majority of the victim population were aware of the importance of the care provided in the**

They were considered to be the best centre for the proper treatment of rabies, given the lack of the necessary equipment in basic health care centres.

2.7. The day of arrival for vaccination:

In our study, the majority of participants (54%) arrived for vaccination on the day of the bite (D0), whereas in another study carried out in Abidjan, more than (50%) of participants arrived after 5 days of the incident [25].

c:> **The high percentage of people who were vaccinated on the same day as being bitten, as reported by the victim population, showed that they were aware of the importance of getting treatment quickly to ensure better and more effective care.**

2.8. Washing the wound :

In our study, 56% of participants did not wash their wounds. This is similar to the study carried out in Abidjan, where 60% of the participants questioned did not wash their wounds. In the same study (Abidjan), for those who did wash their wounds, the product most commonly used was alcohol for no more than two minutes (64%). However, we found that the majority used water with Marseille soap (52%) for a maximum of 5 minutes [25].

c:> **Neglecting to wash and disinfect the wound, the first essential step in treating a bite, may be responsible for the emergence of cases of rabies. With regard to the product used for washing, it is essential to was not inadequate and the duration was insufficient. All these factors can influence the quality of rabies management.**

2.9. Follow-up vaccination after the bite :

With regard to post-bite vaccination booster follow-up, most of our participants had taken all the recommended doses according to the vaccination calendar (43%), whereas the study carried out in Bamako showed that the majority of participants had not followed up on post-exposure vaccination (80%). [22]

The rest of our participants (42%) explained their non-attendance by the following reasons: irresponsibility (41%), lack of transport (34%) and workload (25%). However, in a study carried out in Cotonou, 260 participants interviewed gave the following explanations: lack of transport (70%), workload (15%), no stated reason (15%). [24]

c:> **A percentage of the victim population not vaccinated was quite important, which gives us a vision of the importance of the victim's responsibility to complete all the stages of the rabies control protocol.**

2.10. Veterinary visits:

In the Bamako study, 51.2% of participants took the animal to the vet, which was also in line with our results where the percentage was around 53%. [22]

c:> **We can conclude that there is an awareness of the importance of vaccinating rabies-transmitting animals in order to limit the chain of transmission and prevent the emergence of new cases.**

2.11. Mandatory declaration of rabies :

Among 235 survey participants in the city of Cotonou, more than half (55%) did not consider rabies to be a notifiable disease [24]. In our study, however, we found that the majority (88%) were aware of the obligation to report any confirmed case of rabies.

c:> **According to these results, the subjects surveyed were aware of the seriousness of rabies and considered it to be a notifiable health problem, in order to take action and prevent the risk of an epidemic, but also to analyse the evolution of this disease over time and adapt public health policies to the needs of the population.**

4. Nursing role in rabies prophylaxis :

-Nurses, as health workers, have a vital role to play in preventing rabies by raising the awareness of the target population through :

► Encourage the public to vaccinate transmitting animals, which is the most cost-effective strategy for preventing rabies in humans, as it interrupts transmission at source. In addition, vaccination of dogs reduces the need for post-exposure prophylaxis.

► Inform adults and children about behaviour and clinical signs suggestive of rabies in mammals and how to prevent bites. This is an important step towards ensuring the efficiency of rabies vaccination programmes and reducing the incidence of rabies in humans, as well as the financial burden of treating bites. -To combat rabies by better educating the target population about the first steps to be taken following an attack by an animal capable of transmitting rabies, by reinforcing the community's knowledge of rabies in terms of its characteristics, mode of transmission, clinical signs in humans and animals, the first line of action to be taken and the importance of these steps in promoting the success of the care circuit.

-Ensuring appropriate management by applying the rabies control protocol, while complying with predefined rules and recommendations to minimise the risk of failure.

5. Strengths and limitations :

a) Strengths:

-The main strength of our study lies in its originality. There are not many studies in Tunisian literature that have focused on the knowledge of nurses and victims of animal bites and rabies.
-Rabies is a real health problem that is often underestimated and neglected by healthcare professionals, especially when it comes to human rabies.
-The rate of participation and response to the questionnaires seems to show that the interest shown in this subject by patients and nurses alike.
- For victims, we have translated the questionnaire into Arabic, which improves the relevance of the results, as participants can take their time answering the questions.
- In terms of raising awareness, we have produced brochures and posters containing all the information you need to prevent rabies.

b) Limitations:

-Because of the short duration of the study, we were able to collect 75 bite victims and 80 staff. The interpretation and generalisation of the results to all Tunisian health professionals must be carefully discussed, since our study was not sent to all health professionals.
- In our study, the survey focused on victims only and not on the rest of the population.
- Our sample contained an unequal distribution of men and women.
- The data in our study was completed by the participants themselves, and this may represent a bias that is common in this type of study. However, this bias was minimised by the anonymous and confidential nature of our study.

6. The recommendations :

❖Following our study of rabies at the university hospital, military hospital and basic health centres in Gabes, we offer the following suggestions for reducing the risk of catching rabies:
:> When a person has been in contact with a suspect animal of being rabid, the

nurse must collect the following data:

o The circumstances of the incident:

- provoked or unprovoked
- where it took place, etc.

- the names of other people who may have come into contact with the animal.

o Type of animal :

- wild animal: fox, wolf

- pet: dog, cat.

o Type of contact :

- with saliva, blood, etc.

- biting, scratching, licking, etc.

o If the animal is a pet :

- owner's name

- previous immunisation of the animal

:> To be effective, the various control measures must be based on the following:

▪ Stepping up rabies control in dogs.

▪ Raising awareness among the public and owners of domestic carnivores outside World Rabies Day.

▪ Educating people to monitor the health of their pets.

▪ Educating children about the risk behaviours to be avoided in the workplace. Presence of domestic animals through in schools and colleges.

:> We are also proposing to produce brochures and posters in the health centres and hospitals to raise awareness and insist on prevention.

Rabies is a zoonosis that can affect all warm-blooded animals. Man is an accidental victim, usually as a result of being bitten, scratched or licked on a wound by a rabid animal. It is characterised by an often long incubation period, encephalomyelitis, which is generally fatal, and signs of excitement, aggression and paralysis. Nurses have a vital role to play in the management of rabies, which means they need to be fully trained and up to date with the latest developments in vaccination and protocol to minimise the risk to the community. The lack of equipment is a problem encountered in our study that threatens the successful execution of the protocol as required, which implies urgent intervention in collaboration with the Ministry of Health to compensate for the shortcomings. The victim population is the second most important partner in effective preventive or curative care, and their knowledge has a major influence on the success or failure of interventions. As a preventive measure, rabies vaccination is the only way to protect patients against this disease.Fighting rabies requires collective and individual awareness, as well as effective and ongoing multi-sectoral collaboration within the framework of the national and regional committees, in order to raise public awareness and reduce the incidence of human rabies.

BIBLIOGRAPHY

[1] Kharmachi, H. Hammamis S. Epizoototogy and major zoonoses. Evolution of l'enzootie et de l'endémie rabique en Tunisie. BE IV 1992; 1.

[2] Tlili B. Etude de la répercussion de la compagne de lutte antirabique 1982-1987 sur l'incidence de la rage animale et humaines en Tunisie. Thesis, Faculty of Medicine, Tunis 1988.

[3] Ministry of Public Health. Direction des soins de Santé de base. Unité des anthropozoonose. Programme national de lutte contre la rage, Sidi thabet, 28-29 June 1993.

[4] Aubry P., Rotivel Y., 2001. Infectious diseases Rabies. MédChir; 76 : 320-3.

[5] Toma B, Dufour B., 2007, Rabies, Polycopy of the Contagious Diseases Units of the French Veterinary Schools.

[6] TektoffJ.,Dura four M., Fargeaud D., Précausta P., Souleot J. P., 1982.ComparativeImmunology, Microbiology and InfectiousDiseases5 (1-3), 9-19.

[7] Collard L., 2006. Apport de la biologie moléculaire à la taxinomie et à l'épidémiologie des virus rabiques (Thesis). Médecine Vétérinaire; Lyon 171p.

[8] Ousmane KM, 2010. Contribution à l'épidémiologie de la rage humaine dans les localités urbaines du Mali (Thesis). Médecine Pharmacie et OdontoStomatologie: Bamako; 53p.

[9] Aubry P., Rotivel Y., 2001. Infectious diseases Rabies. MédChir; 76 : 320-3.

[10]Hagos G.W., Muchie F.K., Gebru G.G., Mezgebe G.G., Reda A.K., Dachew A.B., 2020. Assessment of knowledge, attitude and practice towardsrabies and associatedfactorsamonghouseholdheads in

[11] Blancou J, Aubert M, Tsiang H, Bruyère, Masson V ., 2004. Contagious diseases: rabies. French National Veterinary School; 63p.

[12]Natakesuma IK G, Sumantra IP, Grace D, Unger F, Gilbert J., . 2015. On dogs, people, and a rabies epidemic: resultsfrom a socioculturalstudy in Bali, Indonesia. Infectious Diseases of Poverty;4:30.

[13] Smith, A. (2017). Nurses' knowledge and practice in rabies prevention: a systematic review. Journal of Infection Control and Prevention, 15(2), 34-49.

[14] Mohammadi TM, YazdaniCherati J, Shahraki Pour S, et al. "Assessment of nurses' knowledge, attitudes and practices on rabies disease in Morocco." Archives of Clinical Infectious Diseases. 2019 ;14(3) .

[15] Brisseau-Gimbert V, Bourdeau-Quintard B, Delisle C. "Training nurses in rabies risk management: a survey of nursing schools in France." Public Health. 2017 ;29(6) :885-893.

[16] article

[17] Al-Rabiaah A, Ibrahim AK, Al-Ayedh NK. "Effectiveness of rabies awareness posters in improving knowledge and attitudes among healthcare professionals in a tertiary care hospital in Saudi Arabia." Journal of Infection and Public Health. 2020;13(2):304-308.

[18] Agence nationale de sécurité du médicament et des produits de santé (ANSM). "Guide to good practice on the prevention of rabies in humans." Saint-Denis: ANSM, 2016.

[19] 4Public Health Agency of Canada. "Guidelines for the prevention and control of rabies in humans and animals in Canada." Ottawa: Public Health Agency of Canada, 2016.

[20] Garg S, Gupta S, Garg VK, et al. "Modified rapid fluorescence assay for outbreak inhibition and direct fluorescent antibody assay for potency determination of rabies vaccines." Indian Journal of Medical Microbiology. 2016; 34(1): 53- 57.

[21] Sudarshan MK, Madhusudana SN, Mahendra BJ, et al. "Assessment of the burden of human rabies in India: results of a national multicenter epidemiological survey." International Journal of Infectious Diseases. 2007;11(1): 29-35.

[22] Yannick, M. T. (2013-2014). Thesis about human rabies in the infectious diseases department of the CHU de point G A Bamako.

[23] Guesmi K, Kalthoum S, Fatnassi N, Gharbi R, et al (2021). Evaluation of household knowledge, attitudes and practices in relation to a case of human rabies in El-Alia.

[24] Josué, O. M. (2019-2020). Evaluatioon of knowledge, attitudes and practices of Cotonou populations on rabies.

[25] Issaka T, Diloma M, Yao K, Joseph B, et al (2009). Compliance with rabies vaccination in rabies-susceptible individuals in Abidjan (Ivory Coast). p. 595-603.

PERSONAL QUESTIONNAIRE

We are Béni Hamed Abir and Harabi Raouia, two students in their 3rd year at the Institut Supérieur des Sciences Infirmières in Gabes. As part of our end-of-studies work entitled
"'Study of the knowledge of nurses and victims of animal bites with regard to rabies: preventive measures"'.
We would ask you to take part in the development of our survey and to complete this questionnaire objectively and accurately, in the knowledge that all the data collected will be anonymous and confidential.

I. Identifying the study population :

1. Gender :

- Male □
- Female □

2. Age :

- 25-30 □
- **31-40□**
- Over 40 □

3. Length of service :

- <5 years □
- Between 5-10 years □
- >10 **years□**

4. How long have you worked in this department?

- <5 years □
- 5 years and **over□**

5. Which hospital department do you work in?

- Emergency department □
- CSSB □
- Infectious Diseases Department □

II. Study of nurses' knowledge of rabies:

1. Have you had any previous training on the national rabies control programme?

- No □
- Yes □
- If yes: since when and at which centre?

2Is the choice of protocol the responsibility of the :

- Doctor □
- Nurse □
- Doctor and nurse together □

3Have you managed a case of human rabies?

- Yes □
- No □

III. Study of the degree of implementation of a rabies control protocol :

1. Is there a written rabies control protocol posted in your health facility?

- Yes □
- No □
- If not: how do you execute the protocol?
  - ► By memory □
  - ► Contact the doctor in charge □
  - ► Look for the protocol on social networks □
  - ► Other:

2. does your healthcare establishment have the necessary resources to apply

Correct rabies control protocol:

- Yes □
- No □
- If not: what is missing?

3. What is your level of compliance with the rabies control protocol?

• **90%**□

• **50%**□

• Depending on the conditions □

• **Non-respect**□

4. What obstacles have been encountered despite the availability of the necessary resources?

• Workload □

• Incomplete information on rabies □

• Lack of staff □

• Other:

5. What is the first thing to do in the event of an animal bite?

6. Do you wash bites first?

• No □

• Yes □

• If yes: how long does it take to wash?

• What product should you use to wash bites?

7. Do you do the Besredka test before infiltration?

• Yes □

• No □

• IF yes, give the definition of this test:

8. What should you do if the patient is allergic to rabies serum?

► Do not infiltrate □

► Go undercover □

► Admit the patient to the intensive care unit and carry out the **infiltration**□

9. **The infiltration is done**:

• Totally in MI □

• Around wound only □

• Around wound and remaining amount in **IM**□

10. If the bite is located in a sensitive or highly innervated area (eyes, genitals, etc.), do you do the infiltration?

- Yes □
- No □

11. If the wound is large, do you suture it?

- **Yes□**
- No □
- If not, when is thesuture ?

IV. Study of preventive measures

1. Do you provide patient education?

- **Yes□**
- **No□**
- If so: what are the educational themes?

2 . What do you do if vaccination is delayed?

- Nothing to do, it's not my responsibility □
- Call the patient to alert them and start the protocol □
- Other

QUESTIONNAIRE FOR VICTIMS

We are Béni Hamed Abir and Harabi Raouia, two students in their 3rd year at the Institut Supérieur des Sciences Infirmières in Gabes. As part of our end-of-studies work entitled

"'Study of the knowledge of nurses and victims of animal bites with regard to rabies: preventive measures"'.

We would ask you to take part in the development of our survey and to complete this questionnaire objectively and accurately, in the knowledge that all the data collected will be anonymous and confidential.

I. SOCIO-DEMOGRAPHIC DATA:

- Age (years): 18-30□30-35□ 35years or more□
- Sex: Male□Female □
- Geographical origin: Urban□Rural □
- Level of education:Illiterate□Primary□Secondary□University□
- Profession:Yes □No □

If yes, please specify: Student□Executive□Middle manager □
Worker□ Liberal profession □

- Socio-economic level:Low□Medium □High □

II. Study of the knowledge of the victim population about rabies :

1. According to your knowledge, is rabies a fatal disease?

- Yes □
- No □

2. Who can transmit rabies?

- only the dog □
- other mammals □

3. Can humans transmit rabies?

- Yes □
- No □

4. Can I catch rabies from a licked object? by a rabid animal?

- Yes□
- No □

5. Which of these signs suggests the presence of rabies?

- Behaviour change □
- Disturbance of consciousness leading to coma□
- Sensation of burning, tingling instead of biting □
- Difficulty breathing and swallowing. □
- a fear of water (hydrophobia) □
- All proposals are possible □

6. What is your first-line response to a bite? d'unanimal suspected of being rabid?

7. Which centre do you go to first in the event of an animal bite?

- Emergency department □
- A basic healthcare centre (CSSB) □
- A general practitioner □
- No direction on the first day □

8. How long does it take to be seen after a bite?

- J0
- Between D1 andJ4
- Between D4and D7
- Between D7 and D14

9. Do you wash the wound immediately?

- Yes□
- No □
- If yes: which product?
- If so, how long does the wash take?

10. Are you following the vaccination schedule?

- Yes □
- No □
- If not: why not?

11. If you have a pet (dog, cat, etc.), do you visit the vets as required?

•Yes □

•No □

12. Is rabies a notifiable disease?

•Yes □

•No

SUMMARY

Title: Study of nurses' and animal bite victims' knowledge of rabies: preventive measures

Introduction: Rabies is a vaccine-preventable viral zoonosis that affects the central nervous system. Once clinical symptoms appear, rabies is fatal in virtually 100% of cases. As a result, nurses need to reassess their knowledge of rabies and the quality of care they can provide to people attacked by animals that transmit the disease. They also need to process the information acquired from the victim population about the basics they need to know about rabies in terms of what to do, which can influence a well-defined care pathway.

Objectives: the aim of this work is to study the knowledge of nurses and victims of animal bites with regard to rabies, to improve care techniques and therapeutic methods in the emergency department and to propose preventive measures to limit possible complications.

Materials and methods: This was a cross-sectional descriptive study of health personnel working at Gabès University Hospital. In addition, another questionnaire was sent to victims of animal bites in the same health establishments.

Results: Our survey included a sample of 80 staff working in the regional hospital of Gabès, the military hospital and the basic health care centres (Tbelbou, Wassit, Kattena, cité Al'Amal, Manara, Ghanouch and Bouchamma). The sex ratio was 0.6, with women predominating (54%). 80% of the staff questioned had not received training in the national rabies control programme. Furthermore, (32%) of the nurses surveyed did not have a rabies control protocol poster in their health establishments. We therefore concluded that the majority of staff (66%) were unaware of Our study included 75 animal bite victims. The majority of patients interviewed were male (64%), with a sex ratio (M/F) of 2.84. We found that the majority of the victim population (73%) thought that rabies was a fatal disease. More than half (61%) agreed with the possibility of catching rabies through contact with an object licked by a rabid animal.

Conclusion: Nurses have a vital role to play in the management of rabies, and this necessarily involves thorough and complete training. They need to be up to date with the latest developments in vaccination and protocol, to minimise the risk to the community. The victim population is also the second most important partner in effective care. So combating rabies requires collective and individual awareness, and effective multi-sectoral collaboration.

Key words: Rabies, **rabies vaccine, knowledge, nurses, knowledge of victims, prevention measures.**

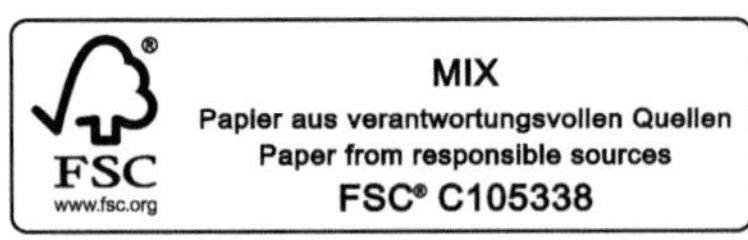

Printed by Books on Demand GmbH, Norderstedt / Germany